MOMS, MILK, AND MIRACLES

Your Guide to Breastfeeding Success

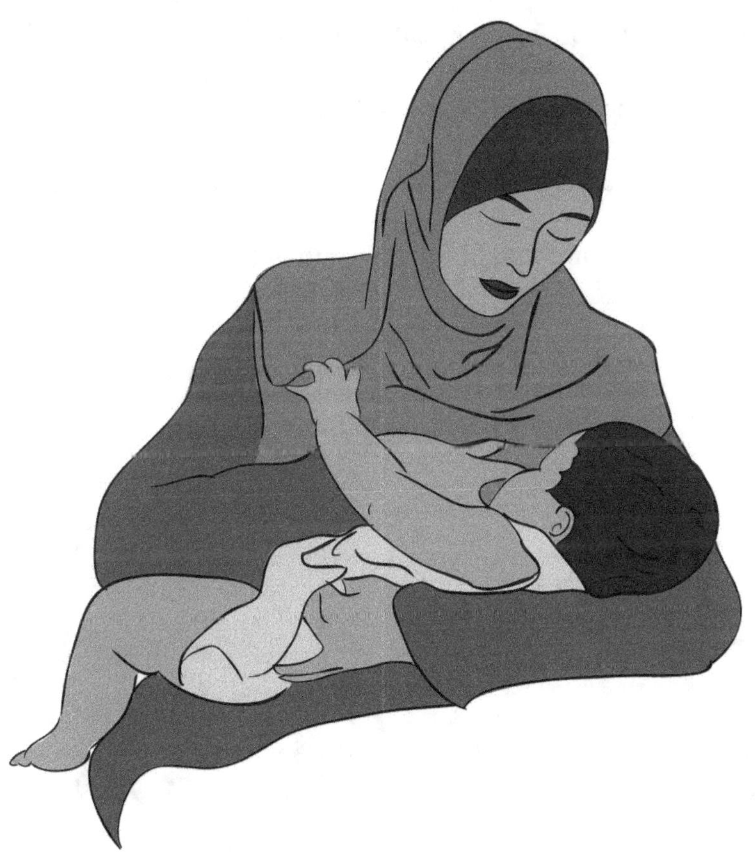

Table of Contents

Foreword

In the realm of parenthood, there exists a profound and transformative journey—a journey woven with the threads of love, sacrifice, and unwavering dedication. At the heart of this odyssey is a beautiful and intimate act: breastfeeding.

Welcome to "Moms, Milk, and Miracles: Your Guide to Breastfeeding Success." This book is an exploration of one of the most significant chapters in the narrative of motherhood. It is a heartfelt tribute to the miracle that unfolds when a mother cradles her newborn child, offering sustenance and affection in a timeless dance of nature.

The act of breastfeeding is a tapestry of countless moments, each a thread binding a mother to her child. It is a testament to the human body's remarkable ability to nurture and protect life. Within the pages of this book, you will embark on a voyage into the world of breastfeeding—a world where science meets love, and the result is nothing short of miraculous.

This journey is not merely a guide; it is a celebration of the bond between a mother and her child, a bond forged through the nurturing embrace of breastfeeding. Here, we delve into the art and science of breastfeeding, exploring the countless benefits it offers to both mother and baby.

Together, we will discover the nutritional excellence of breast milk, providing not just nourishment but also immune-boosting, growth-promoting elixirs. We will explore the emotional connection, the nurturing of a baby's mind and soul, and the empowerment that a mother experiences when she cradles her child at her breast.

This book is a comprehensive resource, a guide through the labyrinth of questions, challenges, and joy that accompanies the breastfeeding journey. It encompasses the essential aspects of preparing for breastfeeding, achieving a comfortable latch, and navigating common hurdles. It addresses nutrition, offering insights into how to best fuel both you and your baby. We'll also touch on the practicalities of pumping, safe milk storage, and how to confidently nurse in public.

Moreover, "Moms, Milk, and Miracles" delves into the stories of success, real-life experiences of mothers who have embarked on this journey, and the wisdom they've gained along the way.

Breastfeeding is a personal and profound journey. As you read these pages, remember that your story is unique and beautiful. The path you walk may be filled with moments of elation, moments of challenge, but, above all, moments of wonder. Whether you are an expectant mother preparing for the arrival of your child, a new mother navigating the early days of breastfeeding, or a seasoned mother embarking on another nursing journey, this book is your guide, your companion, and your source of wisdom.

So, embrace this journey. Savor every moment. Celebrate the bond that breastfeeding creates, the health it nurtures, and the joy it brings. May "Moms, Milk, and Miracles" serve as your beacon of inspiration and empowerment on this incredible voyage.

With love and admiration for the remarkable journey you are about to undertake,

[John D. Lawler]

Chapter 1: The Benefits of Breastfeeding

Breastfeeding is a remarkable and natural way for mothers to nourish their babies, providing numerous benefits for both the infant and the mother. It is a fundamental aspect of early child development, offering a multitude of advantages that go beyond simple nutrition. In this chapter, we'll explore the many reasons why breastfeeding is considered the gold standard for infant feeding.

Nutritional Excellence

Breast milk is often described as "liquid gold" for a good reason. It is a perfectly balanced source of nutrition that meets all the dietary needs of a newborn. Breast milk contains a dynamic blend of essential nutrients, antibodies, and growth factors that adapt to the baby's changing requirements. It is rich in proteins, fats, carbohydrates, vitamins, and minerals, all tailored to promote healthy growth and development. Additionally, colostrum, the first milk produced after birth, provides the newborn with vital antibodies that protect against infections.

Immunological Advantages

One of the most remarkable benefits of breastfeeding is its immunological protection. Breast milk is teeming with immune-boosting components, including antibodies and white blood cells, which shield the baby from a myriad of infections and illnesses. It helps in building the baby's immune system, reducing the risk of respiratory infections, gastrointestinal diseases, and ear infections. Breastfed infants are also less likely to suffer from severe conditions like pneumonia and necrotizing enterocolitis.

Optimal Brain Development

Breastfeeding is not only nourishment for the body but also fuel for the brain. The essential fatty acids found in breast milk, particularly docosahexaenoic acid (DHA), play a crucial role in brain development. Studies have shown that breastfed children often perform better on intelligence tests and exhibit enhanced cognitive development compared to formula-fed infants. The emotional bonding that occurs during breastfeeding also promotes healthy brain development by fostering a secure attachment between mother and child.

Digestive Health

Breast milk is gentle on a baby's delicate digestive system. It is easily digested, reducing the risk of constipation and diarrhea. Breastfed infants are also less prone to food allergies and intolerances. The healthy bacteria present in breast milk and passed from mother to child contribute to the development of a robust gut microbiome, which plays a pivotal role in overall health.

Lifelong Health Benefits

The advantages of breastfeeding extend well beyond infancy. Studies have shown that breastfed babies have a reduced risk of developing chronic health conditions later in life. They are less likely to become obese, have a lower risk of type 2 diabetes, and exhibit decreased rates of certain cancers. Furthermore, breastfeeding is associated with better dental health, as it reduces the risk of dental caries in childhood.

Emotional Connection

Breastfeeding is not solely about nourishment; it's a powerful emotional bond between mother and child. The skin-to-skin contact and the act of breastfeeding create a deep sense of security, comfort, and love for the baby. This emotional connection between mother and child lays the foundation for a healthy emotional and psychological development.

Convenience and Cost-Efficiency

Breastfeeding is remarkably convenient and cost-effective. There are no bottles to sterilize, no formula to buy, and no worries about running out of supplies. It's readily available at the perfect temperature, and it reduces the risk of foodborne illnesses that can sometimes occur with formula feeding.

In conclusion, the benefits of breastfeeding are both numerous and profound. It offers unparalleled nutritional content, immunological protection, and contributes to the overall well-being of both mother and child. It fosters a lifelong foundation of health and emotional connection, making breastfeeding one of the most beautiful and impactful experiences in the journey of motherhood. Whether for a few months or several years, breastfeeding can leave a lasting, positive imprint on a child's life.

Chapter 2: Getting Started with Breastfeeding

The journey of breastfeeding is a remarkable one, beginning even before your baby is born. It's a journey that's filled with love, bonding, and the creation of a profound connection between you and your child. However, like any journey, it requires some planning and preparation. In this chapter, we will delve into the essential steps to get started with breastfeeding, ensuring a smooth and successful initiation.

1. Prenatal Education

The journey of breastfeeding begins during pregnancy. Prenatal education is your first step. Attend breastfeeding classes, read books, and seek online resources to gain a solid understanding of what to expect. These resources will introduce you to breastfeeding techniques, positions, and the many benefits it offers to both you and your baby. Being well-informed before your baby arrives can significantly reduce anxiety and increase your confidence in the process.

2. Create a Comfortable Space

One of the first practical steps you can take is to create a comfortable and inviting space for breastfeeding. Find a cozy chair or nursing station where you can relax. Keep essential items within arm's reach, such as water, snacks, burp cloths, and nursing pads. This setup will be your sanctuary for countless moments of connection with your baby.

3. Choose the Right Nursing Bra

Investing in a comfortable and well-fitting nursing bra is crucial. A nursing bra provides easy access for breastfeeding and offers much-needed support. You may want to purchase a few different styles to see what works best for you, as comfort and fit can vary from person to person.

4. Latching and Positioning

Achieving a proper latch and comfortable positioning for both you and your baby is fundamental to successful breastfeeding. Before you start, make sure you are comfortable and relaxed. Hold your baby close to you, aligning your baby's nose with your nipple. Wait for a wide open mouth, and then bring your baby to your breast. The key is to ensure that your baby latches onto both the areola and the nipple to get enough milk efficiently.

5. Skin-to-Skin Contact

Skin-to-skin contact immediately after birth is invaluable. It not only promotes bonding but also encourages your baby to latch effectively. Let your baby rest on your chest, skin against skin. The warmth and familiarity help establish a connection that will last throughout your breastfeeding journey.

6. Be Patient and Persistent

In the initial days, breastfeeding may not always be smooth sailing. Be patient with yourself and your baby. It's a learning process for both of you. Your baby may need time to adjust and become proficient at latching.

Seek support from a lactation consultant or a healthcare provider if you encounter challenges or have concerns.

7. Feed on Demand

Newborns typically need to feed often, sometimes as frequently as every 1-3 hours. Feed your baby on demand, which means offering the breast whenever your baby signals hunger. This frequent feeding not only satisfies your baby's nutritional needs but also helps establish your milk supply.

8. Trust Your Instincts

Remember that every mother-baby pair is unique. Trust your instincts and listen to your baby's cues. Your baby will let you know when they are hungry and when they are satisfied. As you become attuned to each other, you'll find your rhythm in this incredible journey of nourishment and bonding.

Getting started with breastfeeding is an exciting and sometimes challenging phase. With knowledge, preparation, and patience, you are setting the stage for a beautiful and rewarding journey. As you and your baby navigate the path of breastfeeding, you'll find that it's not just about nourishing your child; it's about creating a lifetime of loving moments and enduring connections.

Chapter 3: Latching and Positioning: The Cornerstones of Successful Breastfeeding

In the intricate ballet of breastfeeding, latching and positioning are the choreography that sets the stage for a harmonious and nourishing connection between mother and baby. Achieving a proper latch and comfortable positioning is essential for a successful breastfeeding journey. In this chapter, we will explore the significance of latching and positioning, offering you insights, tips, and techniques to ensure a smooth and rewarding breastfeeding experience.

The Importance of a Good Latch

A good latch is the key to successful breastfeeding. It ensures that your baby is effectively extracting milk from your breast while minimizing discomfort for both of you. When your baby latches properly, it means they are attached to both your nipple and the surrounding areola. This ensures that your baby gets a good mouthful of breast tissue, allowing for efficient milk transfer and a reduced risk of nipple pain or damage.

Signs of a Good Latch

A proper latch is characterized by:

- Your baby's mouth is wide open, like a yawn.
- The lips are flanged outward, creating a seal around the areola.
- The baby's chin and nose are touching the breast.
- You hear or see swallowing as your baby feeds.

Steps to Achieving a Good Latch

Positioning: Before latching, ensure you and your baby are in a comfortable position. Use pillows or cushions to support your body. Your baby should be facing your breast, and you should hold your breast with your free hand.

C-Hold: Create a "C" shape with your hand, placing your thumb on top and your fingers below your breast. This will support your breast while keeping your fingers away from your baby's mouth.

Tickle the Lips: Gently stroke your baby's upper lip with your nipple. This encourages your baby to open their mouth wide.

Aim for the Mouth: When your baby opens their mouth wide, move your baby towards your breast so that their chin and lower lip touch your breast first. This allows for a deeper latch.

Observe the Latch: Ensure your baby's mouth covers a large portion of your areola. You should see more areola above your baby's mouth than below it.

Comfortable Positions for Breastfeeding

Positioning is as crucial as latching for a successful breastfeeding experience. Various breastfeeding positions allow you to find the one that's most comfortable for you and your baby. Some common positions include:

Cradle Hold: This classic position involves holding your baby in your arm with their head resting on your elbow.

Football Hold: In this position, you tuck your baby under your arm like a football. It's useful for mothers who had a cesarean section or for tandem nursing twins.

Side-Lying Position: This position allows you to lie on your side with your baby facing you, making nighttime feedings more comfortable.

Cross-Cradle Hold: Similar to the cradle hold, but you use the opposite arm to support your baby. This can be helpful for guiding your baby's latch.

Laid-Back Nursing: In this position, you recline in a comfortable chair or bed, and your baby lies on top of you, allowing them to latch at their own pace.

Remember that the choice of position is highly personal. What matters most is that both you and your baby are comfortable and that the latch is effective.

In conclusion, latching and positioning are the foundational elements of a successful breastfeeding journey. The right latch ensures efficient milk transfer and minimizes discomfort, while comfortable positioning allows for relaxed and enjoyable feedings. Seek support from a lactation consultant if you encounter challenges, and trust in the unique bond you are building with your baby through this nurturing act. As you and your baby master the art of latching and positioning, you'll create a beautiful, unbreakable connection that lasts a lifetime.

Chapter 4: How to Increase Milk Supply

Breast milk is nature's perfect food for your baby, and a robust milk supply is crucial for a successful and fulfilling breastfeeding experience. But what if you find your milk supply isn't meeting your baby's needs or you simply want to ensure an ample supply? In this chapter, we'll explore various strategies and techniques to help you increase your milk supply and nurture the beautiful journey of breastfeeding.

Understand Normal Milk Supply

First, it's essential to understand that the volume of milk a mother produces can vary from person to person. Factors such as genetics, hormonal balance, and breastfeeding practices play a role. Normal milk supply is usually established within the first few weeks, and it is influenced by frequent breastfeeding, effective latching, and your baby's demand.

1. Frequent Nursing

The foundation for a healthy milk supply is frequent nursing. The more your baby breastfeeds, the more signals your body receives to produce milk. Newborns often need to nurse every 1-3 hours. As your baby grows, their feeding pattern will evolve, but regular nursing remains vital for maintaining and increasing your supply.

2. Effective Latching and Emptying the Breasts

A good latch ensures that your baby efficiently removes milk from your breasts. When your baby breastfeeds, they start with the thinner, thirst-quenching foremilk, and then progress to the richer hindmilk. Ensuring your baby empties one breast before switching to the other encourages the production of hindmilk, which is rich in fats and calories.

3. Skin-to-Skin Contact

Skin-to-skin contact promotes a strong bond with your baby and encourages breastfeeding. This practice helps your baby feel secure and connected, which can lead to more effective and frequent nursing sessions.

4. Pumping and Hand Expression

Expressing milk through pumping or hand expression can help stimulate milk production. Pumping after or between feedings can mimic your baby's nursing pattern and signal your body to produce more milk. Consider using a double electric breast pump for maximum efficiency.

5. Nutrition and Hydration

A well-balanced diet with plenty of fluids is essential. Staying hydrated and consuming a variety of nutritious foods can help your body generate an adequate milk supply. Some mothers find that certain foods, such as oats, can naturally boost milk production.

6. Rest and Relaxation

Stress can negatively affect your milk supply. Adequate rest and relaxation are essential for maintaining a healthy supply. If possible, nap when your baby naps and ask for help from friends and family to reduce your stress levels.

7. Galactagogues

Galactagogues are substances that can help increase milk production. Some herbal options include fenugreek, blessed thistle, and milk thistle. Consult with a lactation consultant or healthcare provider before using any herbal remedies.

8. Consult a Lactation Consultant

If you're concerned about your milk supply, don't hesitate to seek the guidance of a lactation consultant. These experts can provide personalized advice, support, and strategies to enhance your breastfeeding journey.

9. Nursing on Demand

Allow your baby to nurse on demand. Respond to their cues, even if it means more frequent feedings. This helps establish a strong milk supply tailored to your baby's needs.

10. Keep Baby Close

Proximity to your baby is a powerful signal to your body to produce milk. Consider babywearing, co-sleeping (following safe guidelines), or simply having your baby close by as much as possible.

Remember that the key to increasing your milk supply is patience and consistency. Your body is designed to produce the milk your baby needs. By following these strategies, you can nurture your breastfeeding journey and ensure an ample supply for your growing baby. Enjoy the bonding, nourishing, and comforting moments that breastfeeding provides while building a strong

connection that will last a lifetime.

Chapter 5: Burping Your Baby After Feeding: A Gentle Act of Care

Feeding your baby is not just about nourishing their tiny body; it's a beautiful, bonding experience that allows you to connect on an intimate level. Yet, as every parent knows, it's not just about what goes in; it's also about what comes out. Burping your baby after a feeding is an essential practice that can ensure their comfort and well-being. In this chapter, we'll explore the art of burping, why it's important, and the various techniques to make this process smooth and enjoyable for both you and your little one.

The Importance of Burping

Burping is essential for babies, particularly during and after feeding, because it helps expel air that may have been swallowed while nursing. Infants are still mastering the coordination of swallowing, sucking, and breathing, so it's common for them to ingest small amounts of air during feeds. If this trapped air isn't released, it can lead to discomfort and possibly colic or gas pains.

When to Burp Your Baby

It's crucial to burp your baby during and after each feeding. How often you should burp your baby depends on the baby's age and how they are feeding. If your baby is bottle-fed, burping can be more frequent, as babies tend to swallow more air from a bottle. Breastfed babies may need to be burped less often, but it's still essential to help prevent discomfort.

Signs That Your Baby Needs to Burp

Fussiness or Restlessness: If your baby seems fussy or uncomfortable during or after a feeding, it might be a sign that they need to burp.

Spitting Up: Frequent spitting up or regurgitation of milk can indicate the presence of trapped air.

Gassiness: Excessive gassiness or frequent passing of gas can be a sign that your baby needs to burp.

Burping Techniques

There are several methods to burp your baby, and it's a good idea to try different ones to see which works best for your little one. Here are the most common burping techniques:

1. Over-the-Shoulder: Place your baby over your shoulder with their head resting on your chest. Support their bottom with your hand and gently pat or rub their back. This technique is ideal for newborns and young infants.

2. Sitting on Your Lap: Sit your baby on your lap in a slightly upright position with their chest against your hand. Support their chin with one hand and pat or rub their back with the other.

3. Face-Down on Your Lap: Lay your baby face-down on your lap with their head turned to one side. Gently pat or rub their back. Ensure your baby's face is not covered.

4. Upright Position: Hold your baby in an upright position on your lap with their chin resting on your shoulder. Pat or rub their back gently.

5. Lying Down: Place your baby on their back in a crib, playpen, or a safe, flat surface and gently rub or pat their back. This method is suitable for older babies who can roll over.

Tips for Burping Success

Be patient: Some babies burp easily, while others take more time. It's essential to be patient and gentle during the process.

Use a gentle touch: Avoid vigorous patting or hitting on your baby's back. Use a gentle, rhythmic motion.

Experiment with positions: Try different burping positions to find the one that works best for your baby.

Keep a burp cloth handy: Sometimes, a little spit-up accompanies burping. Having a cloth nearby can help keep both you and your baby clean and comfortable.

Stay calm and relaxed: Your baby can sense your mood. Burping should be a soothing experience for both of you.

In Conclusion

Burping your baby is more than a simple act of releasing trapped air; it's a moment of care and connection. It's an opportunity for you to soothe and comfort your little one, reinforcing the bond that you share. Remember that every baby is unique, so take your time to learn your baby's preferences and needs when it comes to burping. As you establish a routine, you'll find that burping becomes not just a practical necessity but also a cherished part of the feeding experience, one that creates beautiful moments in your shared journey.

Chapter 6: Pumping and Storing Breast Milk: A Mother's Guide to Convenience and Flexibility

Breast milk is a precious gift that nourishes and nurtures your baby, and breastfeeding is a unique and intimate experience. However, there are times when you may need to be away from your baby or want to share the feeding responsibilities with your partner or caregiver. Pumping and storing breast milk offers you the flexibility to provide your baby with the best nutrition, even when you're apart. In this chapter, we will explore the art of pumping and storing breast milk, ensuring you can maintain the breastfeeding journey with ease and convenience.

Why Pump and Store Breast Milk?

Pumping and storing breast milk serves several important purposes:

Feeding on Demand: Pumped milk allows your baby to be fed by a caregiver while you're away, ensuring they receive the nourishment they need.

Relieving Engorgement: If your breasts become uncomfortably full, pumping can relieve pressure and prevent issues like mastitis.

Returning to Work: For working mothers, pumping and storing breast milk is a valuable way to continue breastfeeding while being apart from your baby during the day.

Increasing Milk Supply: Regular pumping sessions can help stimulate and maintain milk production, ensuring a consistent supply for your baby.

Choosing a Breast Pump

There are various types of breast pumps available, and the right choice depends on your specific needs. *Here are some common types of breast pumps:*

Manual Breast Pump: These are simple, hand-operated pumps ideal for occasional use or for mothers who prefer a more straightforward device.

Single Electric Breast Pump: A single electric pump is convenient for occasional use and provides more efficient pumping than manual options.

Double Electric Breast Pump: These pumps are efficient and suitable for daily use, especially for working mothers who need to pump frequently.

Hospital-Grade Breast Pump: Hospital-grade pumps are designed for frequent, long-term use and are often used by mothers with specific breastfeeding challenges.

Pumping Tips

Before you start pumping, consider these tips to ensure a successful experience:

Choose a Comfortable Location: Find a quiet, comfortable place to pump where you can relax. You might want to use a privacy screen if needed.

Warm Compresses: Applying a warm compress to your breasts before pumping can help stimulate milk flow.

Breast Massage: Gently massaging your breasts before and during pumping can help with milk flow.

Use the Right Pump Setting: Start with a low suction setting and gradually increase it to a level that is comfortable and effective for you.

Pump Both Breasts Simultaneously: If you're using a double electric pump, it's more time-efficient to pump both breasts at the same time.

Pump for 15-20 Minutes: Aim to pump for 15-20 minutes per session or until your breasts feel soft and emptied.

Storing Breast Milk

Proper storage of breast milk is essential to ensure its safety and quality. *Here are some guidelines for storing breast milk:*

Containers: Store breast milk in clean, food-grade containers, such as bottles or breast milk storage bags.

Labeling: Label the containers with the date of expression so you can use the oldest milk first.

Hygiene: Wash your hands before handling breast milk, and ensure that all equipment and containers are thoroughly cleaned.

Refrigeration: Freshly pumped breast milk can be stored in the refrigerator for up to 3-5 days at 32-39°F (0-4°C).

Freezing: Breast milk can be safely frozen for up to 6-12 months at 0°F (-18°C). Use a deep freezer for longer storage.

Thawing: To thaw frozen breast milk, place it in the refrigerator or hold it under warm, running water.

Never Refreeze: Once breast milk is thawed, it should be used within 24 hours and should never be refrozen.

Feeding from Stored Milk

When it's time to feed your baby from stored milk, make sure to:

- Use the oldest milk first (first in, first out).

- Gently swirl the container to mix the fat that may have separated during storage.

- Warm the milk by placing the container in warm water.

- Do not use a microwave, as it can create hot spots.

In Conclusion

Pumping and storing breast milk offers a world of possibilities for mothers, from enabling you to return to work while still providing the best nourishment for your baby to allowing others to participate in feeding and bonding. It's a practice that requires a bit of planning and organization but can greatly enhance your breastfeeding journey. By selecting the right pump, following proper pumping techniques, and adhering to storage guidelines, you can ensure that your baby continues to benefit from the priceless gift of your milk, no matter where you are or what your schedule demands.

Chapter 7: Overcoming Common Challenges in Your Breastfeeding Journey

Breastfeeding is a beautiful and natural way to nourish your baby while fostering a deep bond between mother and child. However, it's not always a seamless journey. Many mothers encounter challenges along the way that can make breastfeeding seem like an uphill battle. In this chapter, we will address common breastfeeding challenges and provide guidance on how to overcome them, ensuring that your breastfeeding experience remains a fulfilling and rewarding one.

1. Sore Nipples

Sore nipples are a common challenge in the early days of breastfeeding. This discomfort often arises from an improper latch. *To overcome sore nipples:*

- Ensure a proper latch by seeking guidance from a lactation consultant.

- Allow your nipples to air dry after feedings.

- Use lanolin cream or breast milk to soothe and protect your nipples.

2. Engorgement

Engorgement occurs when your breasts become overly full, making them hard and painful. To overcome engorgement:

- Nurse frequently to help drain your breasts.

- Use warm compresses or take a warm shower before feeding to help milk flow.

- If your baby can't latch due to the firmness, express milk manually or with a breast pump until your baby can latch comfortably.

3. Low Milk Supply

Low milk supply can be frustrating, but there are ways to increase your milk production:

- Ensure a proper latch and frequent nursing sessions.

- Use breast compressions while nursing to increase milk flow.

- Add pumping sessions between feedings to stimulate more milk production.

- Stay hydrated and maintain a balanced diet.

4. Plugged Ducts

A plugged milk duct can lead to localized pain and a lump in the breast. To overcome plugged ducts:

- Continue breastfeeding from the affected breast, focusing on different nursing positions.

- Apply warm compresses before nursing to help clear the duct.

- Massage the affected area during feedings.

5. Mastitis

Mastitis is a painful breast infection that can lead to flu-like symptoms. To overcome mastitis:

- Continue breastfeeding from the affected breast, ensuring proper latch and drainage.

- Rest and stay hydrated.

- Use warm compresses and over-the-counter pain relievers as recommended by your healthcare provider.

- If symptoms persist, consult a healthcare professional for antibiotic treatment.

6. Thrush

Thrush is a fungal infection that can affect both mother and baby. To overcome thrush:

- Treat both you and your baby with prescribed antifungal medications.

- Sterilize or replace pacifiers, bottle nipples, and breast pump parts.

- Maintain good hand hygiene and wash bras and nursing pads regularly.

7. Oversupply of Milk

An oversupply of milk can be overwhelming and lead to engorgement and fast milk flow, making it challenging for your baby to latch. To overcome an oversupply:

- Nurse your baby from one breast per feeding to help regulate milk production.

- Use breast compressions during nursing to control the flow.

- Pump just enough to relieve engorgement, but not to fully empty the breast.

8. Nipple Confusion

Nipple confusion can occur when introducing bottles or pacifiers too early. To overcome nipple confusion:

- Delay introducing bottles and pacifiers until breastfeeding is well-established.
- Select bottles with a slow flow nipple to mimic breastfeeding.

9. Returning to Work

Returning to work while breastfeeding can be a challenge. To overcome this, consider:

- Pumping and storing milk before returning to work.

- Creating a pumping schedule at work and communicating your needs to your employer.

- Using a high-quality breast pump for efficient pumping sessions.

10. Teething

When your baby begins teething, they may sometimes bite during nursing. To overcome this challenge:

- Pay attention to your baby's cues and remove them from the breast if they bite.

- Offer a teething toy or cold washcloth before nursing to soothe their gums.

In Conclusion

The breastfeeding journey is filled with joy, connection, and the benefits of mother's milk. However, it can also present challenges. By addressing common breastfeeding difficulties head-on, seeking support from a lactation consultant, and implementing effective strategies, you can overcome these obstacles and continue to provide your baby with the best nourishment and love. Remember that each breastfeeding journey is unique, and by persisting through these challenges, you are creating a lasting bond and nurturing your child's well-being.

Chapter 8: Nutrition for Nursing Mothers: Nourishing You and Your Baby

The journey of motherhood is a remarkable one, filled with love, joy, and the profound act of nurturing your newborn through breastfeeding. The power to provide your baby with the best possible start in life lies in your milk. Proper nutrition is the cornerstone of a successful breastfeeding experience. In this chapter, we will delve into the crucial role of nutrition for nursing mothers, offering guidance on what to eat, how to maintain your own well-being, and how to ensure that your baby receives the optimal nourishment.

The Importance of Proper Nutrition

Breast milk is a complete source of nutrition for your baby, providing them with the ideal balance of macronutrients, vitamins, minerals, and antibodies to support their growth and development. Therefore, it's crucial for nursing mothers to focus on their own nutritional needs to ensure that the breast milk they produce is of the highest quality.

Caloric Needs

Nursing mothers require more calories to meet the increased energy demands of producing milk. On average, you may need an additional 300-500 calories per day, but individual requirements vary. Listen to your body and eat when you're hungry.

Hydration

Staying hydrated is essential for maintaining milk supply. Aim to drink plenty of water throughout the day.

While there's no specific quantity that fits all, pay attention to your body's signals for thirst.

Nutrient-Rich Foods

A balanced diet is key. Focus on incorporating a variety of nutrient-rich foods into your meals, including:

Protein: Lean meats, poultry, fish, eggs, dairy, legumes, and nuts provide essential protein for muscle and tissue repair.

Complex Carbohydrates: Whole grains like brown rice, whole wheat, and oats supply energy and fiber.

Healthy Fats: Include sources of healthy fats like avocados, nuts, seeds, and olive oil to support brain and eye development in your baby.

Fruits and Vegetables: A rainbow of fruits and vegetables ensures a wide range of vitamins and minerals. Dark, leafy greens are excellent sources of iron.

Dairy or Dairy Alternatives: Milk, yogurt, and cheese provide calcium for bone health. If you're lactose intolerant or following a plant-based diet, choose fortified dairy alternatives.

Fatty Fish: Salmon, mackerel, and sardines are rich in omega-3 fatty acids, which are beneficial for your baby's brain development.

Supplements

In some cases, nursing mothers may require supplements to meet their nutritional needs:

Vitamin D: Breastfed babies may need a vitamin D supplement. Consult your pediatrician for recommendations.

Iron: If your iron levels are low, your healthcare provider may recommend iron supplements.

Prenatal Vitamins: Continue taking prenatal vitamins to fill any nutrient gaps in your diet.

What to Avoid

While nursing, it's important to be mindful of what you consume. Limit the following:

Caffeine: Excessive caffeine can affect your baby's sleep patterns. Limit your caffeine intake and watch for signs of fussiness or difficulty sleeping in your baby.

Alcohol: If you choose to consume alcohol, do so in moderation, and time it appropriately to allow your body to metabolize it before breastfeeding.

Allergenic Foods: If your baby has shown signs of food sensitivities, consider eliminating common allergens like dairy, nuts, or eggs from your diet and reintroduce them one at a time to identify the cause.

Listening to Your Body

Every mother's body and breastfeeding journey are unique. Pay attention to how your body responds to different foods. If you notice that certain foods cause discomfort in your baby, such as gas or fussiness, consider eliminating them temporarily to see if it makes a difference.

Meal Planning and Timing

A regular eating schedule can help maintain your energy levels and milk supply. Plan nutritious meals and snacks throughout the day. Including protein in your meals can help stabilize your blood sugar and prevent energy crashes.

Self-Care

Remember that taking care of yourself is equally important. Try to get enough sleep, reduce stress, and engage in light physical activity when you can. A well-balanced diet and self-care are essential for maintaining both your own well-being and your baby's health.

In Conclusion

Nutrition for nursing mothers is not just about the food you eat; it's about the love and care you provide to your baby. Your body is a remarkable source of nourishment for your child, and it's essential to support it with a balanced and nutritious diet. By focusing on your own nutritional needs and listening to your body, you are not only providing the best start in life for your baby but also ensuring that your breastfeeding journey is filled with

health, happiness, and love.

Chapter 9: Nursing in Public: Embracing Confidence and Empowering Choices

Breastfeeding is a natural and beautiful act of nurturing your baby, and one of the most intimate connections you can share. However, there may be moments when you need to breastfeed in public, which can sometimes raise questions and concerns. In this chapter, we will explore the art of nursing in public, focusing on the importance of confidence, the legal rights of breastfeeding mothers, and practical tips for a comfortable and discreet experience.

The Importance of Nursing in Public

Breastfeeding in public is about more than just feeding your baby; it's about normalizing and celebrating the act of providing the best possible nourishment. It's a public acknowledgment that breastfeeding is a natural and essential part of motherhood. Here are several reasons why nursing in public is vital:

Bonding: Nursing in public allows you to create a deep, intimate bond with your baby wherever you go.

Nutrition: It ensures that your baby gets the nourishment they need, regardless of location.

Independence: It offers the freedom to maintain your lifestyle, engage in social activities, and travel with your baby.

Empowerment: It empowers you to educate and enlighten others about the benefits and beauty of breastfeeding.

Legal Rights of Breastfeeding Mothers

In the United States, there are laws to protect the rights of breastfeeding mothers:

Federal Law: The "Break Time for Nursing Mothers" provision in the Fair Labor Standards Act (FLSA) requires employers to provide reasonable break time and a private, non-bathroom space for nursing employees to express milk.

State Laws: Many states have additional laws protecting a mother's right to breastfeed in public. Research your state's laws to understand your rights and any additional protections in place.

Confidence and Comfort

Nursing in public often becomes easier with experience and confidence. Here are some tips to help you feel more comfortable and self-assured:

Practice at Home: Start by nursing in front of a mirror or with a trusted friend or family member present to help you gain confidence.

Wardrobe Choices: Wear clothing that makes breastfeeding easier. Invest in nursing bras, tops, or dresses designed for easy access.

Using a Nursing Cover: Nursing covers can provide extra privacy, and there are many stylish options available. However, they are not required.

Confidence is Key: Remember that you have the legal right to breastfeed in public. You're giving your baby the best start in life, and you should be proud of it.

Discreet Nursing Techniques

Here are some practical techniques to make nursing in public more discreet and comfortable:

Find a Comfortable Location: Look for quiet spots where you can sit and feed your baby without feeling rushed or crowded.

Use a Scarf or Blanket: You can use a lightweight scarf or blanket to provide some privacy while nursing.

Wear Layers: Wearing layers can allow you to lift your top layer and use your bottom layer as a cover while nursing.

Nursing Pads: Invest in high-quality nursing pads to prevent any leaks from showing through your clothing.

Master the Latch: A proper latch is essential for discreet nursing. Ensure your baby latches well to minimize exposure.

Educating and Advocating

While nursing in public is about your comfort and your baby's needs, it's also an opportunity to educate and advocate for breastfeeding. Here are some ways to engage positively with those around you:

Educate Gently: If someone expresses discomfort or curiosity, kindly explain the benefits of breastfeeding and its normalcy.

Join Support Groups: Consider joining breastfeeding support groups, both online and in your community, to connect with other mothers and share experiences.

Advocate for Your Rights: If you ever encounter discrimination or harassment while nursing in public, don't hesitate to assert your legal rights.

In Conclusion

Nursing in public is not just a practical necessity; it's an essential act of motherhood and a celebration of the remarkable bond between you and your baby. By understanding your legal rights, building confidence, and mastering discreet techniques, you can confidently and comfortably breastfeed wherever you go. Embrace the empowering choice to nourish your child naturally and beautifully, while also advocating for the normalcy and benefits of breastfeeding. Your journey as a breastfeeding mother is a remarkable and inspirational one.

Chapter 10: Weaning: Navigating the Transition with Love and Care

Weaning is a significant milestone in the journey of motherhood, marking the gradual transition from exclusive breastfeeding to a more diversified diet. This chapter explores the art of weaning, offering guidance on when and how to introduce complementary foods, understanding your baby's cues, and navigating the emotional aspects of this transformative period.

Understanding the Right Time for Weaning

The timing of weaning can vary from baby to baby, but it's typically recommended to begin introducing solid foods around six months of age. However, keep in mind that every child is unique, and it's essential to watch for signs of readiness. These may include:

Sitting Unassisted: Your baby should have the muscle strength to sit up and support their head.

Loss of Tongue-Thrust Reflex: When your baby is ready for solids, they will no longer automatically push food out of their mouth with their tongue.

Showing Interest: Your baby might display curiosity about the food you're eating, reaching for it or trying to mimic your chewing motions.

Increased Milk Intake: If your baby's milk intake remains high, they might not be ready for solids yet.

They should be willing to reduce their milk consumption as they transition to solid foods.

The First Foods

The introduction of solid foods is an exciting time for both you and your baby. Here are some guidelines to follow as you begin the journey of weaning:

Start with Single-Ingredient Foods: Begin with simple, single-ingredient foods like rice cereal, pureed fruits (e.g., apples or pears), and vegetables (e.g., sweet potatoes or carrots).

Offer Soft Textures: Initially, the texture should be very smooth to avoid choking hazards. As your baby becomes more accustomed to solids, you can gradually introduce thicker textures.

Go Slow and Gradual: Don't rush the process. Start with one meal a day and gradually increase to two or three meals, maintaining milk feedings.

Avoid Allergenic Foods: While introducing solids, consider avoiding common allergenic foods like peanuts and shellfish.

Sippy Cups: Around 6-7 months, you can start introducing a sippy cup with water to help your baby learn to drink from a cup.

Following Your Baby's Cues

Throughout the weaning process, it's important to listen to your baby and be flexible. Some babies take to solids quickly, while others may need more time to adjust. Look for cues such as:

Interest: Your baby should show curiosity about the food you offer and open their mouth when the spoon approaches.

Hunger: Ensure your baby is hungry before offering solids to increase their interest and willingness to try new foods.

Fullness: Pay attention to your baby's cues of fullness, like turning their head away from the spoon or becoming disinterested.

Patience: Be patient if your baby initially rejects certain foods. It may take multiple tries before they accept a new taste or texture.

Balancing Solids and Milk

As you introduce more solid foods, it's essential to maintain your baby's milk intake, as it remains a crucial source of nutrition. Gradually decrease the frequency of milk feedings as your baby becomes more accustomed to solids. Keep in mind that the balance between milk and solids can vary from baby to baby.

Emotional Aspects of Weaning

Weaning is not only a physical transition but an emotional one as well. It can evoke mixed feelings for both you and your baby. Here are some emotional aspects to consider:

Feelings of Loss: You might experience a sense of loss or sadness as the breastfeeding relationship changes.

Independence: Weaning signifies your baby's growing independence, which can be a source of pride and nostalgia.

Emotional Connection: The emotional connection between you and your baby will continue to evolve as you navigate the weaning process.

Bonding through Food: Use this transition as an opportunity to bond with your baby over food. Share mealtimes together and enjoy the process of exploration and discovery.

In Conclusion

Weaning is a natural progression in your baby's development, marked by the introduction of solid foods and a shift in the breastfeeding relationship. As you embark on this journey, remember to be patient, flexible, and attentive to your baby's cues. It's a time of growth, change, and newfound experiences, all filled with love and care. Embrace this transformative period with confidence and enthusiasm, and treasure the beautiful moments that accompany the weaning process.

Chapter 11: The Partner's Role in Breastfeeding: A Crucial Pillar of Support

Breastfeeding is a profound and intimate experience that not only nourishes a baby but also strengthens the bond between mother and child. However, the journey of breastfeeding doesn't solely rest on the mother's shoulders. Partners play an integral role in providing the support, encouragement, and understanding that make breastfeeding a successful and fulfilling experience. In this chapter, we'll explore the invaluable role that partners play in the breastfeeding journey, and how they can contribute to its success.

Understanding the Importance of Partner Support

Breastfeeding, while a natural process, can be physically and emotionally demanding for mothers. Partner support can make a significant difference in the experience. Here's why it's crucial:

Emotional Support: Breastfeeding can be an emotional journey, with ups and downs. Partners provide a vital source of emotional support, helping to navigate the challenges and celebrate the triumphs.

Physical Assistance: Partners can assist with various aspects of breastfeeding, from preparing snacks for the nursing mother to helping with household chores, allowing her to focus on her baby.

Relationship Building: Supporting breastfeeding fosters trust and communication in a relationship. It's a shared endeavor that can strengthen the bond between partners.

Practical Assistance: Partners can help research breastfeeding information, assist with latch issues, and attend breastfeeding classes to learn more about the process.

Educating and Advocating

Partners can become breastfeeding advocates by gaining knowledge about the benefits of breastfeeding and the needs of a breastfeeding mother. Here's how they can help:

Attend Prenatal Classes: Join the mother in prenatal classes that focus on breastfeeding. Learning together can enhance understanding and preparation.

Be Informed: Educate yourself about the nutritional and emotional benefits of breastfeeding for both the baby and the mother.

Provide Encouragement: Offer words of encouragement and praise for the mother's breastfeeding efforts. Acknowledge her dedication and perseverance.

Advocate for Breastfeeding: If needed, help create a supportive environment for breastfeeding, whether in public spaces or among family and friends.

Practical Assistance

Practical help from partners can ease the daily challenges that breastfeeding mothers face. Here are ways partners can provide support:

Nighttime Feedings: Partners can take on some nighttime feedings using pumped breast milk or formula, allowing the mother to rest.

Diaper Changes: Share diaper-changing responsibilities, as changing diapers and breastfeeding often go hand in hand.

Meal Preparation: Assist in meal planning and preparation to ensure the mother has nourishing and convenient meals and snacks.

Household Chores: Take on household chores to reduce the mother's stress and workload.

Running Errands: Offer to run errands, such as grocery shopping, so the mother can stay home and rest or focus on breastfeeding.

Creating a Supportive Environment

A supportive environment at home and among friends and family is essential for breastfeeding success. Partners can contribute to this by:

Educating Others: Share breastfeeding information with friends and family members to encourage a supportive atmosphere.

Set Boundaries: Politely establish boundaries to ensure that the mother has privacy and comfort when breastfeeding.

Communicate Openly: Maintain open communication with the breastfeeding mother about her needs and concerns, and address any challenges as a team.

Emotional Support

Breastfeeding can be an emotional journey filled with highs and lows. Partners can provide the emotional support needed by:

Listening: Act as a listening ear and a shoulder to lean on. Offer empathy and understanding when the mother encounters challenges.

Offering Reassurance: Remind the mother that she is doing an exceptional job and that you believe in her ability to provide for the baby.

Celebrate Achievements: Celebrate milestones and achievements in the breastfeeding journey, such as reaching a certain duration of exclusive breastfeeding.

Share Responsibilities: Ensure the mother has time for self-care and relaxation to prevent feelings of overwhelm and burnout.

In Conclusion

The partner's role in breastfeeding is invaluable. By providing emotional support, practical assistance, and a supportive environment, partners help create a positive atmosphere that fosters breastfeeding success. Remember that breastfeeding is a journey shared between partners, creating a bond that not only nourishes the baby but strengthens the relationship between parents. Through love, understanding, and teamwork, partners can make the breastfeeding journey a fulfilling and rewarding experience for both the mother and the family as a whole.

Chapter 12: Breastfeeding Myths and Facts: Navigating the Truth

Breastfeeding is a beautiful and natural way to nourish your baby while fostering a deep bond between mother and child. However, this journey is often surrounded by various myths and misconceptions that can lead to confusion and unnecessary stress for new mothers. In this chapter, we will debunk common breastfeeding myths and provide the facts, empowering mothers with accurate information to embark on a confident and successful breastfeeding experience.

Myth 1: Breastfeeding Hurts

Fact: While some initial discomfort can occur as your baby latches on, breastfeeding should not be painful.

Pain is often a sign of an improper latch. Seek help from a lactation consultant to ensure a comfortable latch and feeding experience.

Myth 2: Small Breasts Produce Less Milk

Fact: Breast size has no bearing on your ability to produce milk. The amount of milk produced is primarily determined by how well the baby is latched and how frequently you nurse. Even mothers with smaller breasts can produce an ample milk supply.

Myth 3: You Can't Breastfeed If You Have Inverted Nipples

Fact: Many mothers with inverted or flat nipples can successfully breastfeed. Using techniques like the "flipple" or a breast shield can help with latching. Consult a lactation consultant for guidance.

Myth 4: You Must Follow a Strict Diet While Breastfeeding

Fact: While it's essential to maintain a balanced diet for your well-being, breastfeeding mothers don't need to follow a strict diet. In general, you can eat a variety of foods, including your favorites. If your baby has specific food sensitivities, consult a healthcare professional.

Myth 5: Breastfeeding Leads to Saggy Breasts

Fact: The changes in breast shape and size during breastfeeding are primarily due to pregnancy hormones and genetics. The act of breastfeeding itself doesn't lead to significant breast sagging. Wearing a well-fitting, supportive bra can help maintain breast shape.

Myth 6: Formula is Just as Good as Breast Milk

Fact: While formula can provide adequate nutrition, breast milk offers unique benefits. It contains antibodies, enzymes, and nutrients that protect and nourish your baby in ways formula can't replicate. It's the gold standard for infant nutrition.

Myth 7: You Can't Breastfeed if You Smoke or Drink Alcohol

Fact: While it's best to avoid smoking and excessive alcohol consumption while breastfeeding, occasional and moderate alcohol consumption can be compatible with breastfeeding. Smoking is discouraged, but the benefits of breastfeeding still outweigh potential risks if a mother smokes.

Myth 8: Your Baby Needs Water Alongside Breast Milk

Fact: Breast milk is over 80% water, and in most cases, it provides your baby with all the hydration they need. In the first six months, breast milk is sufficient to keep your baby well-hydrated.

Myth 9: Your Baby Needs to Nurse on a Strict Schedule

Fact: Newborns feed on demand. They signal when they're hungry, and it's important to respond promptly. As your baby grows, they may establish a more predictable feeding schedule, but flexibility is key.

Myth 10: You Must Stop Breastfeeding When You Return to Work

Fact: Many working mothers successfully continue breastfeeding. You can pump and store breast milk for your baby while you're apart. Federal laws in the United States protect your right to pump at work.

Myth 11: Breastfeeding Prevents Pregnancy

Fact: While breastfeeding can suppress ovulation and fertility in some women, it's not a reliable method of contraception. It's possible to become pregnant while breastfeeding, so discuss family planning with your healthcare provider.

Myth 12: Breastfeeding is a Source of Embarrassment in Public

Fact: Breastfeeding is a natural and essential act. Many countries have laws protecting a mother's right to breastfeed in public. Confidence and awareness can help mothers comfortably nurse their babies in public spaces.

Myth 13: You Should Stop Breastfeeding When Your Baby Gets Teeth

Fact: Babies often get their first teeth around six months of age. You can continue breastfeeding with appropriate latch and positioning. If your baby bites, gentle discipline and consistent communication can address the issue.

Myth 14: If You Have a Low Milk Supply, You Must Stop Breastfeeding

Fact: Low milk supply can often be addressed through improved latch, increased feedings, and proper breast stimulation. Consult a lactation consultant or healthcare provider for guidance. Breastfeeding can still be maintained.

In Conclusion

Breastfeeding myths can create unnecessary concerns and challenges for new mothers. Armed with the facts, mothers can confidently embrace the breastfeeding journey and experience the joy, bonding, and health benefits it provides. Understanding the truths about breastfeeding empowers mothers to make informed decisions and cherish this unique and natural experience

with their baby.

Chapter 13: Connecting with Other Breastfeeding Moms

Breastfeeding is a beautiful and natural journey that offers both mothers and babies numerous benefits, including a profound bond and essential nourishment. However, this journey can sometimes be challenging, and connecting with other breastfeeding moms can provide invaluable support, advice, and camaraderie. In this chapter, we will explore the significance of connecting with other breastfeeding moms, ways to find support, and the advantages of a supportive community.

The Importance of Connecting with Other Breastfeeding Moms

Breastfeeding can be a transformative experience, filled with joy, questions, and challenges. Connecting with other breastfeeding moms is vital for several reasons:

Shared Experiences: Other breastfeeding mothers can empathize with your journey, offering insight and understanding because they've been through similar experiences.

Advice and Tips: Breastfeeding veterans often have helpful advice, tips, and practical suggestions that can make your journey smoother and more enjoyable.

Emotional Support: Breastfeeding can be emotionally taxing at times, and sharing your feelings with others who understand can provide comfort and reassurance.

Community and Friendship: Building connections with other breastfeeding mothers can lead to lasting friendships and a sense of community.

Where to Find Supportive Communities

There are various places and resources where you can connect with other breastfeeding moms:

Local Support Groups: Many communities have local breastfeeding support groups or La Leche League meetings where mothers can gather to discuss their experiences and seek guidance.

Online Forums and Social Media: Online platforms and social media groups provide an opportunity to connect with a vast network of breastfeeding mothers worldwide. Websites like "KellyMom," "The Bump," and "BabyCenter" have active breastfeeding forums.

Breastfeeding Classes: Attending prenatal or postnatal breastfeeding classes can introduce you to mothers who share your breastfeeding journey.

Mom and Baby Groups: Joining mom and baby groups or playgroups in your area often includes mothers who are breastfeeding and looking for social connections.

Hospital Resources: Hospitals and birthing centers often provide resources and contact information for local breastfeeding support groups and lactation consultants.

Advantages of a Supportive Community

Being part of a community of breastfeeding mothers offers numerous benefits:

Education: You can learn more about breastfeeding techniques, positions, and best practices from mothers who have "been there, done that."

Emotional Resilience: Sharing your joys and challenges with others can provide emotional support, reducing feelings of isolation and boosting your confidence.

Friendships: Building connections with other mothers can lead to meaningful friendships that go beyond breastfeeding discussions.

Problem Solving: When you encounter breastfeeding challenges, a community of experienced mothers can offer practical solutions and advice.

Advocacy: A supportive community can advocate for breastfeeding-friendly environments, helping to normalize breastfeeding for future generations.

Engaging in Supportive Conversations

Connecting with other breastfeeding moms is about more than just sharing experiences. Engaging in conversations that support and uplift one another is essential. Here are some topics to discuss within your breastfeeding community:

Breastfeeding Success Stories: Celebrate your achievements and share stories of successful breastfeeding to inspire and encourage others.

Challenges and Solutions: Talk about your breastfeeding challenges and explore potential solutions together.

Nutrition and Self-Care: Discuss nutrition, self-care practices, and ways to maintain your health while breastfeeding.

Feeding Strategies: Share insights on feeding schedules, introducing solid foods, and transitioning from breastfeeding to other forms of nutrition.

Advocacy: Work together to advocate for breastfeeding-friendly spaces in your community, including restaurants, malls, and public spaces.

In Conclusion

Connecting with other breastfeeding moms is an essential aspect of your breastfeeding journey. A supportive community provides not only practical advice and guidance but also a network of friendships and a source of emotional strength. The bond formed with other breastfeeding mothers is a testament to the beauty of this shared experience, and it can provide an enduring source of support and encouragement for you and your baby.

Chapter 14: Stories of Success: Celebrating Triumphs in the Breastfeeding Journey

Breastfeeding is a profound and beautiful journey that nurtures the connection between a mother and her baby. Along this path, many mothers encounter challenges, but they also experience remarkable successes. In this chapter, we celebrate the stories of success in the breastfeeding journey, highlighting the triumphs, the perseverance, and the deep bonds that emerge as a result.

Story 1: A Journey of Firsts

In the quiet hours of the morning, new mother Sarah cradled her newborn baby in her arms. The soft, dim glow of the nursery nightlight illuminated the tiny face in her embrace. As she carefully guided her baby to her breast, she felt her heart race with excitement and trepidation. The room was filled with the anticipation of firsts—the first latch, the first moments of connection, and the first drops of precious colostrum.

The initial days of breastfeeding were a whirlwind of emotions for Sarah. The challenges were real, and her questions seemed endless. She worried about her baby's weight gain and whether she was producing enough milk. But she persevered. She attended breastfeeding support groups and reached out to lactation consultants for guidance.

As the days turned into weeks, and the weeks into months, Sarah's dedication bore fruit. Her baby grew healthy and strong, all the while thriving on the nourishing gift that only a mother can provide. The first few weeks had been a steep learning curve, but the moments of triumph and closeness were worth every moment of uncertainty.

Story 2: Overcoming Challenges

Breastfeeding can be a beautiful journey filled with warmth and connection, but it's not without its challenges. Lauren knew this all too well when she embarked on her breastfeeding journey with her first child. Painful latches, cracked nipples, and sleepless nights marked the initial days.

However, Lauren was determined. She refused to let these challenges stand in the way of providing her baby with the best nourishment possible. She reached out to a lactation consultant, who helped her with latch techniques and recommended nipple shields to reduce pain. Slowly but surely, the pain subsided, and the moments of bonding and nourishing her baby overtook the earlier difficulties.

Lauren's story is a testament to the power of perseverance. She demonstrated that even in the face of challenging obstacles, a mother's love and determination can pave the way for a beautiful breastfeeding journey.

Story 3: Tandem Nursing

Tandem nursing is a unique and remarkable success story. It's a journey that involves breastfeeding two children simultaneously—often an older sibling and a newborn. Jane, a mother of a toddler and an infant, embarked on this extraordinary adventure.

Navigating the intricate balance of nurturing two children's emotional and physical needs was not without its challenges. Jane found herself nursing her newborn while also comforting her toddler with her other breast. She was amazed by her ability to bond with both children at once, the loving gazes of her toddler and the contented sighs of her newborn.

Jane's story of tandem nursing is a true celebration of love and commitment. She demonstrated that the heart of a mother has an infinite capacity for nurturing and connecting with her children.

Story 4: Extended Breastfeeding

Extended breastfeeding, which continues beyond the first year of a child's life, is a beautiful success story. It's a journey that defies societal norms and celebrates the unique connection between a mother and her child. Emily's experience of extended breastfeeding is a testimony to the enduring bond it creates.

Emily continued to breastfeed her child well into toddlerhood, cherishing the moments of comfort and connection it provided. She faced questions and raised eyebrows from those who didn't understand, but Emily knew that she was providing her child with not only nourishment but also the emotional comfort and security that extended breastfeeding offers.

Her story exemplifies the beautiful success of nurturing a child through breastfeeding, long after the first days of infancy have passed.

Story 5: Breastfeeding and Working

Breastfeeding and working outside the home can be a challenging juggling act. Lily, a determined mother, faced the challenge of returning to work while continuing to breastfeed her baby. She navigated the world of breast pumps, milk storage, and nursing breaks with grace and determination.

Lily pumped at work during her lunch breaks and breaks to maintain her milk supply. She meticulously stored her breast milk and coordinated pick-ups with her caregiver. Her commitment to breastfeeding remained unwavering, and her story serves as an inspiration for working mothers everywhere.

Lily's success story demonstrates that breastfeeding can continue to flourish, even in the face of busy work schedules and competing demands.

Story 6: Relactation and Adoption

Relactation, the process of restarting breastfeeding after a temporary cessation, is a remarkable journey. Rachel, a mother who faced breastfeeding challenges and initially stopped nursing, embarked on the path of relactation.

With the help of a lactation consultant and her determination, Rachel resumed breastfeeding her baby. Her story demonstrates that the power of a mother's love and perseverance knows no bounds.

Another beautiful success story is that of adoption and breastfeeding. Megan adopted a baby and was determined to provide the nourishment and bonding that breastfeeding offers. With dedication, she used various methods to induce lactation and eventually nursed her adopted baby. Her story showcases the infinite possibilities of love and nourishment through breastfeeding.

Story 7: Supporting Each Other

Success stories are not limited to individual experiences. They often involve a community of support. Many mothers find solace in the stories of other breastfeeding mothers who have faced similar challenges. These supportive communities offer a sense of camaraderie and encouragement, making the journey easier for all.

In these communities, mothers share their stories of success and offer advice, comfort, and understanding to one another. They celebrate one another's triumphs, providing a safe space for questions and support. These communities exemplify the power of shared experiences in the breastfeeding journey.

Story 8: The Power of Breast Milk Donation

Breast milk donation is a selfless and beautiful success story that transcends individual experiences. Mothers who generously donate their breast milk to babies in need highlight the compassion and empathy that breastfeeding can inspire.

Lisa's story is one of these selfless acts of love. She became a breast milk donor to help premature babies in the neonatal intensive care unit. Her dedication to pumping and donating breast milk for these fragile infants showcases the incredible power of generosity and the life-giving properties of breast milk.

Story 9: Navigating Cultural and Social Stigma

In some parts of the world, breastfeeding may face cultural or social stigma. Success stories often involve mothers who break down barriers and proudly breastfeed in public, educate their communities about the benefits of breastfeeding, and redefine cultural norms.

Sophia, a mother from a conservative community, encountered cultural resistance to breastfeeding in public. She faced societal expectations that breastfeeding should be hidden away, but she chose to challenge these norms. By openly breastfeeding in public and educating her community about the benefits of breastfeeding, Sophia redefined the cultural perspective on nursing.

Her story is a testament to the courage and determination of mothers who stand up for their right to nourish their babies naturally and without shame.

Story 10: A Journey of Love

Ultimately, the greatest success story in breastfeeding is the profound connection between mother and child. The bond created through breastfeeding is a testament to the love, dedication, and strength of a mother's heart. Each breastfeeding journey is a unique story of love and triumph, filled with its own moments of success and joy.

The journey of love that mothers and babies embark on is the most beautiful success story of all. It's a celebration of the love, connection, and nourishment that breastfeeding provides. Each story is a testament to the unique and profound bond between mother and child that only breastfeeding can offer.

In Conclusion

Breastfeeding is a remarkable journey, a testament to the love, determination, and strength of mothers. The stories of success in the breastfeeding journey remind us of the extraordinary bonds created between mothers and their children. They inspire, encourage, and celebrate the triumphs, both big and small, that come with the beautiful journey of nourishing and nurturing a baby.

Afterword: A Celebration of Love, Nourishment, and Connection

As we come to the end of this book, I hope you have found it to be a source of knowledge, inspiration, and support on your breastfeeding journey. The chapters within these pages have explored the depths of the breastfeeding experience, from the physical aspects of latch and milk supply to the emotional facets of love, connection, and perseverance. Now, as we conclude, I'd like to leave you with a final reflection.

Breastfeeding is a unique and personal journey, and your story is as extraordinary as any you've read within these pages. Whether you are just starting your breastfeeding journey, well into it, or reminiscing about the moments you've shared with your child, remember that this journey is a testament to the love between a mother and her baby.

In the moments of triumph, when you witness your child thriving and bonding with you, and in the moments of challenge when you persevere through pain or doubt, you are nourishing your baby, not only with your milk but also with your love. The breastfeeding journey is a powerful expression of maternal love, dedication, and the profound connection that only a mother and child can share.

As you look back on your journey or prepare for the one ahead, take pride in the dedication, strength, and resilience that you have demonstrated. The stories of success, the shared experiences, and the support you've found in your community are all a testament to the remarkable journey you've undertaken. You are part of a worldwide community of mothers, each with her unique story to tell, and your story is just as inspiring as any.

Let this book be a reminder that you are never alone on your breastfeeding journey. There is a network of support available to you, whether it's through local support groups, online forums, lactation consultants, or simply the loving embrace of friends and family. Embrace this community of support, for it is your source of encouragement and understanding, and it is always here for you.

As you navigate the path of motherhood through breastfeeding, cherish the moments of success, learn from the challenges, and hold dear the bond that you and your baby share. This journey is not just about milk and nourishment; it's about love, connection, and the enduring legacy of a mother's embrace.

The story of your breastfeeding journey is one of love, sacrifice, and beauty. It is a story that continues with every feeding, every gaze between you and your child, and every milestone achieved. It is a story that celebrates the triumphs of motherhood and the profound connection you share with your baby.

Thank you for allowing me to be a part of your journey, and for sharing in the celebration of love, nourishment, and connection that is the essence of breastfeeding. May your story be filled with the joy, success, and love that you and your child so richly deserve.

With warmest wishes and heartfelt congratulations,

[John D. Lawler]